Prospects Training and Development

The Value Base of Social and Health Care

An NVQ-based Open Learning Pack for Social Care Workers

by

NEIL THOMPSON

Prospects Training and Development

Preface

The Author

Dr Neil Thompson is a senior lecturer in social work at the North East Wales Institute of Higher Education. He has previously worked as a social worker, team leader and training officer. Neil is the author of six books:

> *Practice Teaching in Social Work: A Handbook,* (with Martina Osada and Bob Anderson) Pepar Publications, 2nd edn, 1994.

> *Crisis Intervention Revisited,* Pepar Publications, 1991.

> *Existentialism and Social Work,* Ashgate, 1992.

> *Anti-Discriminatory Practice,* Macmillan, 1993.

> *Dealing with Stress,* (with Michael Murphy and Steve Stradling), Macmillan, 1994.

> *Theory and Practice in Health and Social Welfare,* Open University Press, forthcoming.

The Value Base of Social and Health Care is the first in the Fundamentals of Social Care series. Neil is not only the author of the first pack but is also the overall series editor.

Prospects Training & Development

Prospects Training Publications intends to bring together as contributors to an ongoing series of Open Learning, Study and Training materials a range of specialist contributors and writers. The activities of Prospects Training Publications are managed by an Editorial Board.

Contents

Welcome

... to Prospects Training and Development NVQ Training Pack, The Value Base of Social and Health Care. This pack is designed to help you build up the knowledge base you need to do your job to best effect.

We hope that you will find the pack not only interesting and stimulating but also of practical use in your day-to-day work. Indeed, this is the basis of the NVQ philosophy - that there is an underpinning body of knowledge ('critical and enabling' knowledge) that forms a key part of being able to do your job.

The pack is arranged into different sections to reflect the different aspects of NVQ requirements. The introduction spells this out in more detail and also explains how the pack is to be used - as part of a programme of 'Open Learning'. The overall aim is to provide you with the knowledge and information you need in a clear and accessible form. That is, we present what you need to know in a 'user-friendly' form with diagrams, examples and exercises to aid understanding and 'bring the ideas to life'.

The 'Introduction' outlines the contents of the pack and explains how you should use it to gain maximum benefit from the time and energy you will be devoting to your own training and development.

Learning is usually an enjoyable and exciting process. We particularly hope that this pack will play a part in ensuring that you enjoy developing and enhancing the knowledge and skills your job requires.

Introduction

Who is this pack for?

The pack is for social care staff seeking to become qualified at NVQ level 2 or above. It is not a 'training course' in its own right but, rather, a resource for you to use as part of the broader process of learning from your work experience. Perhaps the most important part of your learning is your skill development - that is, increasing your ability to do your job, making the most of your potential. Skill development comes from experience, but experience is not enough on its own if you are to make the most of the opportunities for learning available to you. And this is where the 'underpinning knowledge' comes in. This is the knowledge base you need in order to:

- Know which are the appropriate skills to develop;

- Understand what is expected of you in terms of good care practice;

- Improve your understanding of some of the complexities of social care;

- Appreciate the legal and policy requirements of your job;

- Build up your confidence by helping you develop an informed approach to the difficulties involved in maintaining high standards of social care.

One of the strong points of the NVQ approach to vocational training is that it builds on strengths. You will already be competent in many areas and will already have much of the knowledge you need. In this way, a pack such as this will reassure you about what you already know and help you fill in the gaps in terms of what you do not know.

So, in short, this pack is for those who have some degree of skill and knowledge but are keen to take these forward as part of a process of continuous professional development.

What is Open Learning?

Open Learning is becoming an increasingly popular approach to education and training. The basic idea is that you, the learner, are provided with the information you need, the basic knowledge you need to do your job effectively. This information is provided in text form but often supplemented by diagrams or tables to help make the material more 'digestible'.

Also, to make learning a more active process, we have included a number of exercises for you to carry out - whether alone or jointly with your colleagues. These are designed to help you think through the issues that we raise and be able to apply them to your own work situation. These exercises are not 'tests' or hurdles for you to jump. Rather, they are presented as aids to learning, devices to help make the ideas more concrete and more directly relevant to your work experience. We would therefore strongly encourage you to resist the temptation to 'skip' exercises and move straight on. If you do give in to this temptation, you will miss out on a number of opportunities for broadening and deepening your learning. Also, the exercises are a good way of comparing notes with your colleagues and, in so doing, creating the opportunity for you to learn from each other. One of the advantages of Open Learning is that you can, to a certain extent at least, learn at your own pace. It pays to get into the habit of keeping the pack close to you, whether at home or at work, so that you can use it whenever it suits you. You can 'dip into' the pack when you have a spare half-hour. It really is up to you to find a pattern of study that suits you - Open Learning gives you the flexibility to do this and, we hope, the motivation to want to take every opportunity to make progress with your learning.

Applying theory to practice

One of the long standing problems in social work and social care, as far as training and development are concerned, is what seems to be a huge gulf between theory and practice, an uncomfortably wide gap between formal theoretical knowledge and what actually happens in the day-to-day reality of social care practice. This is an unsatisfactory, and even dangerous, state of affairs:

> *If we fail to see theory and practice as two sides of the same coin, we run the risk of treating them as two almost totally separate entities. This, in turn, leads to social work practice being based on intuition and common sense. Both of these have a part to play but they are clearly inadequate on their*

*own. Intuition cannot offer an understanding of human
motivation, relationships and social organisation or indeed,
of their complex interaction.
(Thompson, 1992, pp. 11-12)*

Unfortunately, many practitioners have, over the years, turned their backs on theoretical knowledge with comments such as: 'I prefer to stick to practice' or 'It's experience that counts, not what you read in books'. Of course, there is an element of truth in both of these statements. As far as the first is concerned, practice is, after all, what it is all about. However, the attitude underlying this type of comment is an unhelpful one as it means that theory is seen as something not connected with practice. As far as the second statement is concerned, it is partly true. It is, of course, experience that counts but theory is not intended to replace experience. On the contrary, it is intended to enhance experience, to help you get as much out of it as possible. Indeed, it is not experience that is of use to us, but rather, what we learn from that experience - and this is where theory comes in, by giving us a framework for learning. Experience that we do not learn from is of little or no value, and can, in some cases, act as a barrier to future learning. This pack, then, represents an attempt to narrow the gap between theory and practice, to present aspects of the knowledge base you need in a way that is clear and accessible, in a way that encourages you to try the ideas out in practice - this is, after all, the most effective way of learning: learning by doing.

What does the pack cover?

The pack is divided into five main sections, each representing an aspect of the value base of social care. In this way, the pack reflects the structure of NVQ Unit O - 'Promote equality for all individuals'. The five sections of the pack are:

1 *Anti-discriminatory practice* This section addresses issues of prejudice, discrimination and oppression and seeks to create a climate of genuine equality of opportunity - for staff and service users alike.

2 *Confidentiality* Here the focus is on understanding rights of control over personal information. Confidentiality is a complex and sensitive issue and so an informed approach is called for.

3 *Rights and choice* Individuals have rights and it is therefore important for staff to understand what these are, how they can be safeguarded and how real choice can be offered.

4 *Individuality and identity* Individual differences, preferences and a sense of identity are important aspects of personal well-being. There are therefore important lessons to be learned in terms of how these matters can best be dealt with.

5 *Communication skills* Effective and appropriate communication is an essential part of good practice. This section therefore covers the basic skills and principles of good communication.

The pack ends with a brief conclusion that draws together the main themes and issues and sets the scene for your future learning. This pack covers a particularly important aspect of practice and one that relates closely to all the other units of competence within the NVQ framework. This is because values have such an important part to play in social care. As the commentary for Unit O puts it:

This is the value base unit. It details in clear criteria the principles of good practice on which all interactions with individuals (not only clients but other workers, colleagues, managers etc.) are to be based. Although all of the other units have the principles of good practice embedded in them, workers and others (such as managers, assessors, verifiers) will need to refer to this unit for a more precise interpretation of the value base. This unit includes more detailed criteria and more extensive knowledge specifications regarding the principles of good practice than are possible in each of the other units. The value base unit is applicable to every other unit in the framework. It is an integral part of every qualification.

This pack should therefore play a vitally important role in helping you move towards your qualification - not only by helping you achieve this unit of competence but also by laying the foundations for other units of competence too. The ground that this pack covers is therefore doubly important. However, before making a start on the main sections of the pack itself, it is worth commenting on what the pack does not cover. It is important that the pack is not comprehensive in its coverage for the following reasons:

- The subject area covered is quite vast and it would take a pack the size of an encyclopaedia to cover it all adequately;

- Aspects of the area's covered will vary from agency to agency, establishment to establishment and so we cannot cater for all eventualities;

- We wish to encourage an active approach to learning, rather than a passive approach based on 'spoon feeding'.

As with any form of learning, what we offer here is part of a broader process. It is to be hoped that the pack will provide you with much of the learning needed as well as the motivation and confidence to continue learning - to build on, and consolidate, the foundations that this pack can help establish.

What do I do now?

You are now ready to make a start on studying the pack. But, before you do, it would be worth spending a few minutes making sure you are clear about:

- Who else is studying this pack? Which colleagues can I rely on for support?

- What time scale am I working to?

- What pace of study suits me best? What are the best times and place for me to study? Am I able to manage my time to good effect?

If you are unclear about any of these, or about any other aspect of working towards your qualification, make sure you talk to your line manager, training officer or a supportive colleague. If you have any problems or anxieties, it is advisable to try and get them sorted sooner, rather than later. Slight anxiety can be a spur to learning but too much anxiety acts as a significant barrier to learning. So, the answer is simple: talk over any anxieties that you may have before they grow out of proportion. So when you're ready, get your brain into gear and away you go!

Anti-Discriminatory Practice

ELEMENT O.a
Promote Anti-discriminatory Practice

Why is anti-discriminatory practice important?

There are three main reasons why anti-discriminatory practice is not just important but actually essential. These are:

1 Discrimination is illegal. Appendix 1 provides details of the legal requirements for equality of opportunity.

2 Discrimination is oppressive and therefore morally unacceptable. We cannot claim to be a caring profession and condone or carry out discrimination and oppression.

3 Anti-discriminatory practice builds on positives. By challenging discrimination we are undermining negative stereotypes and helping to empower people. (Empowerment is an important concept we shall look at in more detail below.)

These, then, are the three primary arguments for anti-discriminatory practice: legal, moral and practical. What they have in common is that they are arguments about good practice. In short, anti-discriminatory practice is good practice. Once we have recognised this, we can then move on and look at how we can ensure that our practice is anti-discriminatory - part of the solution, rather than part of the problem (Thompson, 1993). That is, we can consider how our work can:

a. avoid discriminating against people and
b. challenge and undermine discrimination and oppression more generally.

What is anti-discriminatory practice?

Certain groups in society tend to be treated negatively and subjected to various forms of oppression, whether these be overt and explicit (such as violence or verbal abuse) or more subtle and hidden (such as discrimination against members of ethnic minorities within the housing allocation system see CRE,1985).

Discrimination can apply to any individual or group but certain people tend to be more prone to negative discrimination than others, as Figure 1.1 (below) illustrates. Anti-discriminatory practice is an approach to social care that recognises forms of discrimination and oppression such as racism and sexism and is committed to challenging them. However, this is not simply a matter of dealing with personal prejudice for, as we shall see, discrimination reflects the way society is structured or organised (in terms of class, gender, race/ethnicity and so on). As Webb and Tossell (1991) comment:

> *Caring takes place within a social setting and it is
> important that the significance of this social context is
> understood in order that we, as carers, are able to
> appreciate the impact of the wider society on the
> individual.(p.ix)*

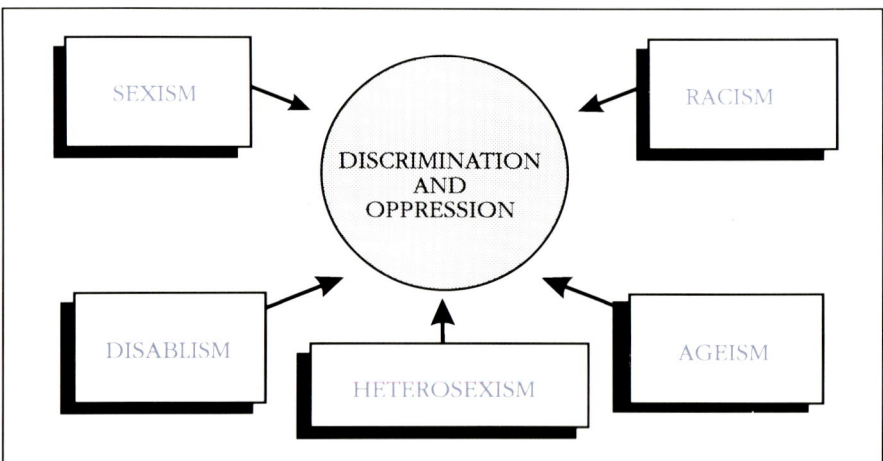

*Figure 1.1
Discrimination
and social groups*

Because discrimination is a social, as well as individual matter, it is not acceptable for us to say 'I am not racist' or 'I am not sexist' as if this absolves us from taking any further responsibility for anti-discriminatory practice. There are four reasons for this:

1 What is important is outcomes, rather than intentions. That is, although there may be no intention to discriminate, the result or outcome may, none the less, prove discriminatory or oppressive. For example, trying to be caring and supportive towards a disabled person may be experienced by the person concerned as patronising and undermining of independence (see Oliver, 1983, 1989);

2 Similarly, we may discriminate without realising that we are doing so, for example, by treating certain people in

a stereo typical way. Indeed, this is how stereotypes tend to work - they lead us into making assumptions and generalisations without realising that this is what we are doing;

3   Discrimination occurs at an institutional level. That is, racism, sexism and so on are not simply personal issues; they are built into the way an organisation or service operates. For example, black children are over-represented in compulsory care yet black families are under-represented in the provision of supportive services. We can therefore detect that there is something discriminatory about the policies or services, rather than the actions of a bigoted minority. Anti-discriminatory practice is not just about our own attitudes and practice, it is also about challenging and undermining the prejudice, discrimination and oppression we encounter in others and in organisations.

Developing anti-discriminatory practice therefore places considerable demands upon us. Let us now consider how we can tackle these issues. We shall begin by exploring the different forms that discrimination or oppression can take.

Recognising oppression

'Oppression' is a term usually associated with tyrannical political regimes However, it is important that we recognise that it also applies on a smaller, more local scale to the actions and attitudes of individuals, groups and organisations. This covers a wide range of examples, as Figure 1.2 illustrates.

These are, of course, not the only ones as the range is quite extensive. Exercise 1.1is designed to help you 'get to grips' with these by relating them to your own experience. Spend a little time now on exercise 1.1 (at the end of this section) before moving on.

Developing sensitivity to oppression and discrimination is a key step in the direction of anti-discriminatory practice. Also helpful in this respect is an understanding of the common forms or categories of discrimination. It is to these that we now turn.

Forms of discrimination

There is no end to the ways in which people can be discriminated against or oppressed. You do not have to be a member of a particular social group to experience the negative effects of prejudice and discrimination. However, it would be naive not to recognise that certain groups in society are exposed to a disproportionate amount of negative attention, for example, women, black, disabled or older people. In this section of the pack we shall look at some of these more common examples of discrimination and consider their implications for social care. We shall look at each of these major forms of discrimination in turn, beginning with issues of gender.

Sexism

Bullock and Stallybrass (1977) define sexism as:

> a deep-rooted, often unconscious system of beliefs, attitudes and institutions in which distinctions between people's intrinsic worth are made on the grounds of their sex and their sexual roles. (p.571)

The major implication of this for social care is that we must be very careful not to reinforce gender stereotypes and thereby assign women and girls to subordinate and less prestigious roles and, in so doing, restrict their opportunities or 'life chances'. A key aspect of this is the language that we use for language is not a 'neutral' reflection of reality - it actively 'constructs' or reinforces that reality. For example, using words like 'chairman' have the effect of excluding and marginalising women. It not only reinforces the notion that 'its a man's world', but also teaches our children to think in these terms, thereby encouraging sexism in future generations. Webb and Tossell (1991) comment on the role of language in perpetuating sexism:

> Language plays a major role in informing us of how society views women and men. There are many aspects of contemporary English language which reveal prejudicial attitudes; for example, the use of pronouns, word order and forms of address. Each helps to reinforce the dominant social values. Everyday language can be seen to support the status quo, i.e. the subjugation of women and the dominance of men. One clear injustice with regard to language is the requirement for females to declare their marital status. Women are addressed as 'Miss' or 'Mrs.'

depending on whether or not they are married, but men, for whom 'Mr.' is the general courtesy title, need not reveal whether they are married. This situation has been mitigated to some extent in the past 20 years with the adoption of the non-specific female courtesy title of 'Ms.' although it is often wrongly used only to describe single women, thereby defeating the point of its intended usage. A further inequality is in evidence when, after marrying, it is the woman who is conventionally expected to surrender her family name and adopt that of her husband. (p. 44)

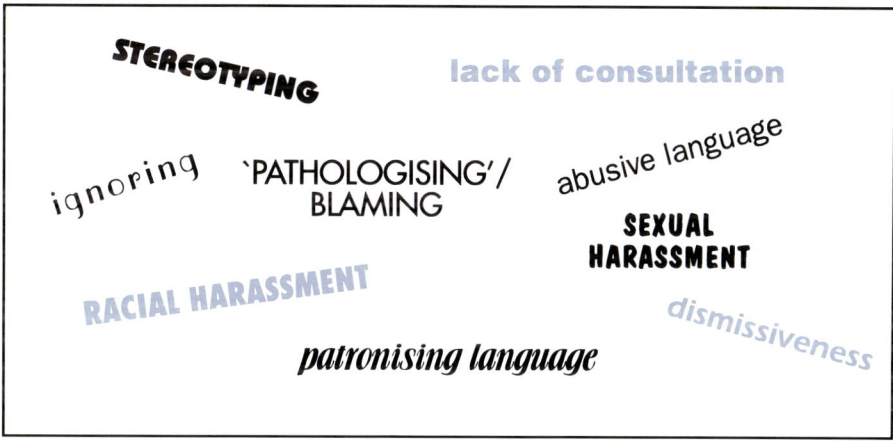

Figure 1.2

Sexism has important implications for social care, especially as the majority of carers, both paid and unpaid, are women. One very significant implication of sexism is its detrimental effect on confidence and self esteem. People are accorded different roles according to their gender - and, in this way, females tend to lose out to males. We therefore have a part to play in making sure that feelings of inferiority are not created or reinforced.

Racism

Lorde (1984) defines racism as 'the belief in the inherent superiority of one race over all others and thereby the right to dominance' (p.115) - and yet the idea of 'races' as distinct biological groups is a false one, an over-simplification of the complexities of human biology. As Husband (1986) comments:

race is not a real entity, whilst racism as a range of personal and institutional practices is very real in its existence and impact. The core of racism consists of people acting as though race concepts were valid criteria for differentiating among human beings; yet there is wide support for the view that there is no adequate biological

EXERCISE 1.1

Consider the examples of oppression given in Figure 1.2. Can you identify situations within your work environment where these may happen? Can you think of other examples of oppression? Use the space below to make some notes.

NB

This is not a test so do feel free to consult your colleagues. Use this as an opportunity to learn from each other basis for believing in 'race' as the idea is so frequently used inBritain.... However, the lack of scientific support for the validity of categorising people into 'races' has done little to undermine the everyday usage of such terms. (p.3)

In a nutshell then, racism arises when we categorise people into assumed biological groups ('races') and then see some groups as inferior. In this way, racism is parallel with sexism - it uses biology as an excuse for differences of power, opportunity and status in society. This can apply at three levels - personal, cultural and structural, as Figure 1.3 (below) illustrates. Once again, this emphasises that racism is not just an individual or personal matter but has much wider and deeper implications.

It is essential for good practice that we do not make assumptions about black and other ethnic minority families and individuals. Or, to use Bandana Ahmad's (1990) term, we must not 'pathologise' black people by seeing them as inferior. Good practice must be:

Ethnically sensitive: by being aware of, and sensitive to, cultural differences between ethnic groups; and -

Anti-racist: by refusing to condone racism and by challenging it whenever and wherever it is encountered.

Figure 1.3
Three levels of racism:
personal, cultural
and structural

PERSONAL	Personal prejudices, negative attitudes and so on.
CULTURAL	Stereotypes, shared assumptions, and values, humour and so on.
STRUCTURAL	Organisational factors, policies and institutional practices.

Disablism

'Disablism' is a relatively new term and was coined to describe the discrimination and oppression experienced by disabled people:

> *Disablism refers to the combination of social forces, cultural values and personal prejudices which marginalises disabled people, portrays them in a negative light and thus oppresses them. This combination encapsulates a powerful ideology which has the effect of denying disabled*

*people full participation in mainstream social life.
(Thompson, 1993, p.105)*

One of the main elements underpinning this is a patronising attitude towards disabled people - patronising in the sense that the emphasis is on 'care' rather than independence. The Disabled People's Movement, a movement that has developed in recent years, is very critical of traditional approaches to people with disabilities. They see disability as a matter of human rights in which the problems disabled people face arise, not so much from their physical impairment itself, but from the way society treats them. For example, the fact that wheelchair users do not have access to certain buildings is a problem caused by the way society operates rather than by any physical impairment. In this way, it can be seen that people with disabilities are, literally, disabled by society. Disability is therefore a social and political issue as well as a personal and individual one. We need to be very careful in ensuring that our work with disabled people involves enabling and empowering them, rather than disabling and oppressing them. We need to avoid the discriminatory stereotypes of disabled people as poor victims of tragedy who need to be 'cared for'. This is where, as we saw before, good intentions are not enough as well-intentioned attempts to be caring and supportive may be experienced as intrusive and oppressive. That is, if we are not careful, we will act in a paternalistic way, perhaps leaving our service users feeling as though they have been treated like children. This does not mean that we should not care - of course we should. It means that our focus must be on providing assistance so that disabled people can look after themselves as much as possible. This is a key aspect of empowerment - giving people more control over their own lives. Very often this will mean trying to remove obstacles to self-care rather than simply being providers of care.

Ageism

Fennell *et al.* (1988) define ageism as: 'the unwarranted application of negative stereotypes to older people' (p. 97). This involves adopting a negative and dismissive approach towards older people, based on a view that they are a burden or a nuisance. This is exemplified by the way old people are so often presented as a figure of fun in comedy programmes on television. Equally ageist is the patronising approach that sees older people as poor unfortunates who need to be looked after. Unfortunately, this is a traditional aspect of social care with elderly people where a medical approach may be adopted. For example, residents in care homes may be described as 'patients' and may have little say in decisions about their care. Here, there is a strong parallel with the description above of disablism where the focus is on doing things for people rather than exploring to what extent it is possible for them to be helped to do things for themselves. Again, we need to foster a sprit of empowerment rather than dependency. Once again, language has a significant part to play. The term, 'the elderly' can be seen as patronising and dismissive, a good example of how older people tend to be dehumanised. We should therefore always remember to add the word 'people' (elderly people) or, better still, use terms such as 'older people' or the more respectful 'elders'. We should also be careful to avoid patronising terms like 'old dear' or 'old darling'. As was emphasised earlier, it is not the good intentions that count when we use such terms, but rather the discriminatory effects or outcomes.

Another example of how language can be discriminatory or oppressive is where older people can be addressed by their first name in situations where younger adults would be afforded the courtesy or respect of a formal title such as Mr. or Mrs. In working with older people we therefore need to make sure that we are not reinforcing stereotypes by adopting a paternalistic approach. We must remember that older people are people first. They are, after all, 'our future selves'. Although the term ageism is generally applied to older people, we can, however, also see its applicability to working with children and young people. We should be wary of stereo typing any group of people according to age. This is likely to lead to far more problems than solutions. For example, if we expect teenagers to be difficult and disruptive just because of their age, then we run the risk of setting up a'self-fulfilling prophecy'. That is, expecting them to be disruptive will actually encourage them to be so.

Heterosexism

This is another relatively newly coined term. It refers to discrimination against people on the grounds of their sexual orientation. It involves seeing lesbian women or 'gay' men as inferior or somehow a threat. In particular, the notion of threat is captured in another important term: 'homophobia', which means fear of homosexuality and contempt for homosexuals. Homophobia and heterosexism often manifest themselves in humour and a view of homosexuality as unnatural or morally wrong. However, from the point of view of anti-discriminatory practice, we need to bear in mind how oppressive such attitudes are:

*The term 'heterosexism' will be unfamiliar to many
because it's fairly new. It has been coined, just as 'racism'
and 'sexism' were coined 'to describe an attitude of mind
that categorises, and then unjustly dismisses as inferior, a
whole group of fellow citizens'. It is institutionalised in our
laws, media, religions and language and in all too many
family 'units'. 'Attempts to enforce heterosexuality are as
much a violation of human rights as racism and sexism
and must be challenged with equal determination'. (GLC,
1985)*

Discrimination against people on the grounds of their sexual
orientation can be seen as oppressive in general terms, but
especially for people in need of social care provision where
discriminatory attitudes can have a profoundly negative effect. The
Children Act 1989 has partially recognised this. For example, the
DOH guidance on family placements states, in relation to
youngsters leaving care, that: 'the needs and concerns of gay
young men must be recognised and approached sympathetically'
(Sone, 1991). One of the major implications of heterosexism is that
we are led into seeing gay men and women largely or solely in
terms of their sexuality. We can fail to see them as whole people.
We can respond in a partial and distorted way and, in so doing,
contribute to oppression and dehumanisation.

Conclusion

Having now considered five of the main forms of discrimination, it
is worth spending some time looking at the 'commonalities' or
common themes that apply across the board. Exercise 1.2 (at the
end of this section) is designed to help you do this.

Developing anti-discriminatory practice is not an easy or
simple task. It involves questioning our own assumptions -
assumptions which may have been reinforced in us over a period
of decades. It also involves challenging others - individuals and
organisations - so that we can genuinely say that our work neither
discriminates nor condones discrimination on the part of others.
Developing anti-discriminatory practice is a long and difficult
undertaking. It is a matter of values - valuing everybody equally,
regardless of who they are or what social group they are part of -
and so it is something we must wrestle with constantly. It is a
process that will continue in the remaining sections of this pack
and, indeed, throughout your NVQ-linked studies where equality

of opportunity and dignity are central themes. Because this is a difficult and demanding process, you may well feel tempted at times to pass it by and just 'get on with the job'. We very much hope that you will be able to resist this temptation. The subtle operation of mechanisms of discrimination and oppression have been ignored and misunderstood for long enough. Now that we are becoming increasingly aware of the workings of discrimination and the destructive impact on significant numbers of people in need of social care provision, it would be a great pity to slow down the progress we are making. So, if you are tempted to give up playing your part, we would urge you to remember three things:

1 Good practice must be anti-discriminatory practice;

2 Discrimination works in subtle and insidious ways. If we are not sensitive to this, we are likely to condone or reinforce oppression without realising it. In short, if we are not part of the solution, we must be part of the problem;

3 You are not alone. Anti-discriminatory practice and values are necessary for all of us. Talk to your colleagues about the issues and share the responsibility together. For anti-discriminatory practice to become a reality, and remain so, a collective effort is needed.

We very much hope that you will be able to play your part in promoting anti-discriminatory values in social care. It will be a difficult process, perhaps painful at times, but we owe it to the people we work with to make it a success.

Important Note

Before moving on to the next section of the pack, just spend a few minutes looking back over this section on anti-discriminatory practice. It is important that you have an overview of these issues clear in your mind before tackling the next set of issues, those of confidentiality.

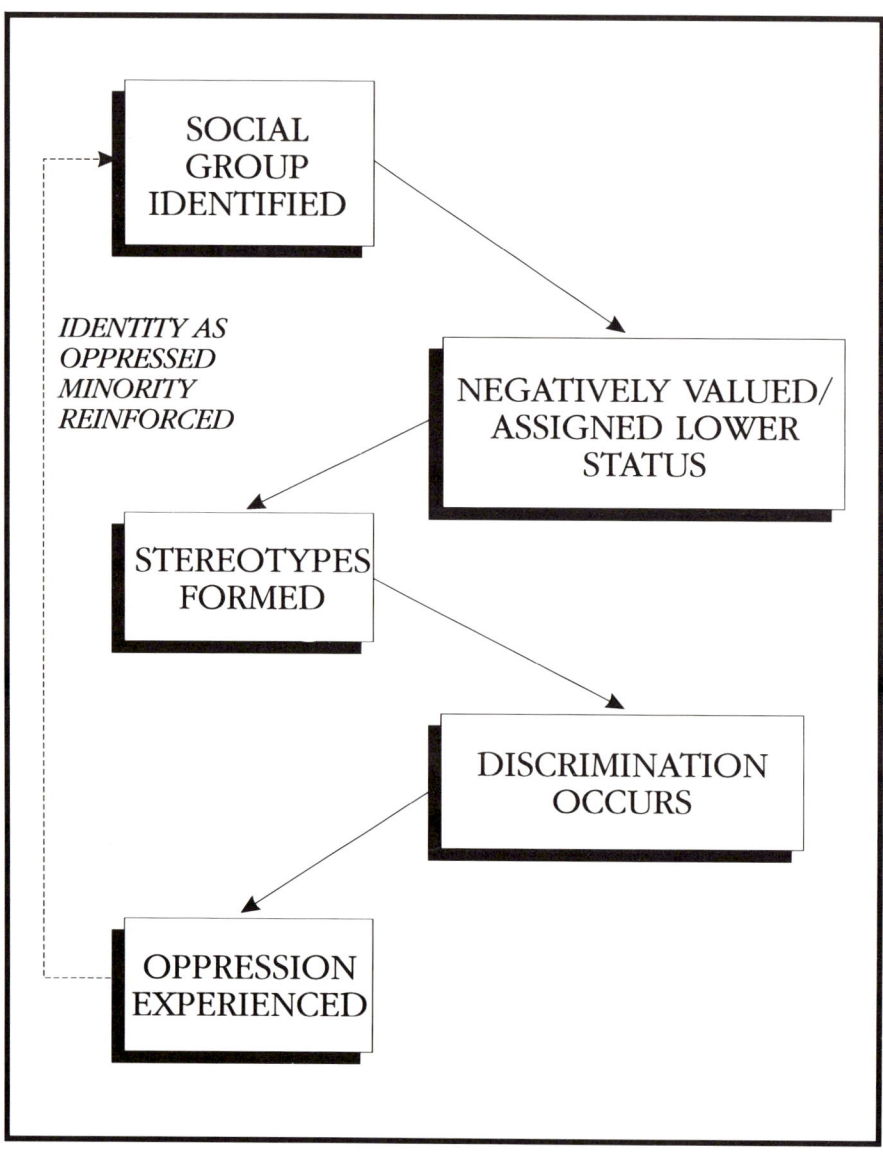

Process of discrimination and oppression

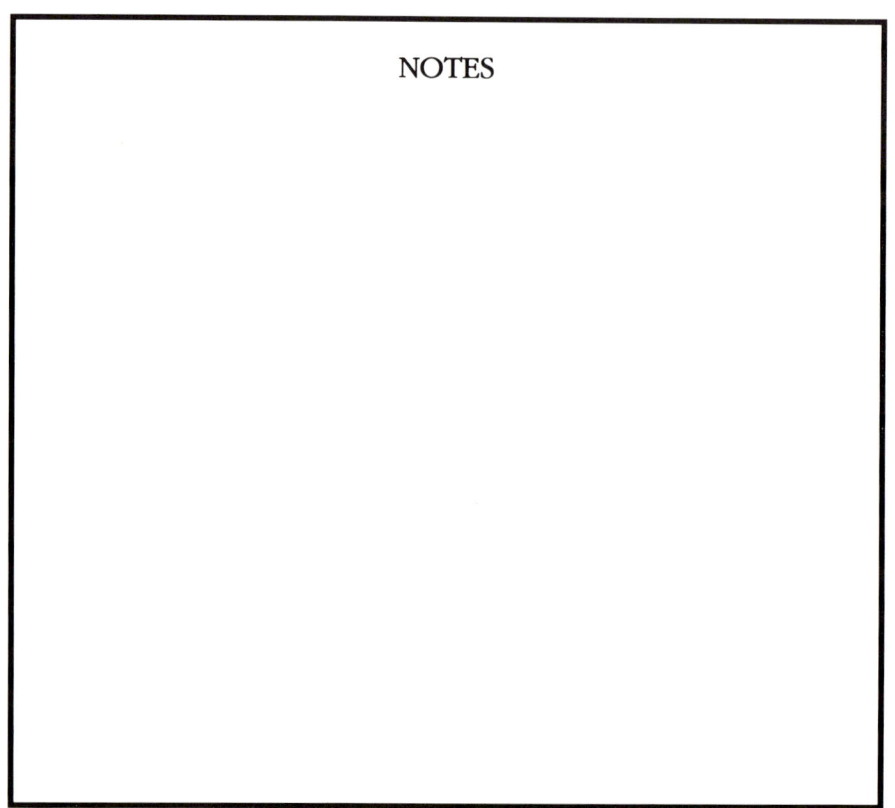

NOTES

EXERCISE 1.2

In developing anti-discriminatory practice there are a number of key terms that we need to understand. Below is a list of some of these key terms that apply across a range of different forms of discrimination. Your task in this exercise is to ensure that you know what they mean (as applied to discrimination and oppression). You can use an ordinary dictionary, a specialist dictionary (for example, a dictionary of sociology), an encyclopaedia or simply discuss them with friends and/or colleagues. How you do it is not important, but what is important is that you do understand what these terms mean.

Once again you should use the space provided to make notes.

stereotype:

prejudice:

power:

equality of opportunity:

ethnicity:

marginalisation:

oppression:

gender:

empowerment:

NOTES

NOTES

2

Confidentiality

ELEMENT O.b
Maintain the confidentiality of information

Why is confidentiality important?

Because we work with information received from clients or from other sources, the way in which we deal with it will have major implications for our relationships with our service users. That is, if information is used carelessly or inappropriately clients are likely to have little trust in, or respect for, staff. They may feel betrayed, used and devalued - not worthy of the privacy and respect they would normally expect to enjoy. Failing to handle information carefully, sensitively and appropriately can therefore have very damaging consequences. It follows, then, that it is important for us to be clear about the 'do's and don'ts' of information so that we can be sure that a lack of confidentiality does not cause problems for our clients, ourselves and our employers. Confidentiality is a fundamental value of social care and so we run the risk of things going badly wrong if we do not take full account of these important issues of confidentiality. To help you with this, this section of the pack looks at some of the key questions that arise in relation to confidentiality. The first one to be tackled is perhaps the most basic one: What exactly do we mean by confidentiality?

What is confidentiality?

Biestek (1961) defined confidentiality as:

> *the preservation of secret information concerning the client which is disclosed in the professional relationship. Confidentiality is based upon a basic right of the client; it is an ethical obligation of the case worker and is necessary for effective casework service. The client's right, however, is not absolute. Moreover, the client's secret is often shared with other professional persons within the agency and in other agencies; the obligation then binds all equally. (p. 121)*

Biestek was referring to casework, the traditional approach to social work, but the same points can be seen to apply also to social care. Let us now look, in a little more detail, at each of these in turn.

1 Secret information

Confidential information is, by definition, secret information; it is not intended to be generally available. This raises the question of boundaries - where do you draw the line between who should know and who should not? - an important point to which we shall return below.

2 A basic right

Like all citizens, people in need of social care have certain basic rights and we need to recognise confidentiality as a primary one amongst these. It is important for people's dignity, self-respect and self-esteem.

3 Not an absolute right

However, in some circumstances, the right to confidentiality may need to be over-ruled, for example, for legal reasons or the protection of others. Once again, we shall discuss this further under the heading of 'boundaries'.

4 Shared information

As care workers, we operate on behalf of an employing agency. Information is therefore confidential not to you as an individual but to your agency - for example in terms of written records. This can sometimes lead to conflicts and dilemmas.

5 Equal obligation

When confidential information is shared within a social care agency or between agencies, it, none the less, remains confidential. The fact that it has been shared to some degree does not mean that it can be shared further - what is shared is the obligation to maintain confidentiality.

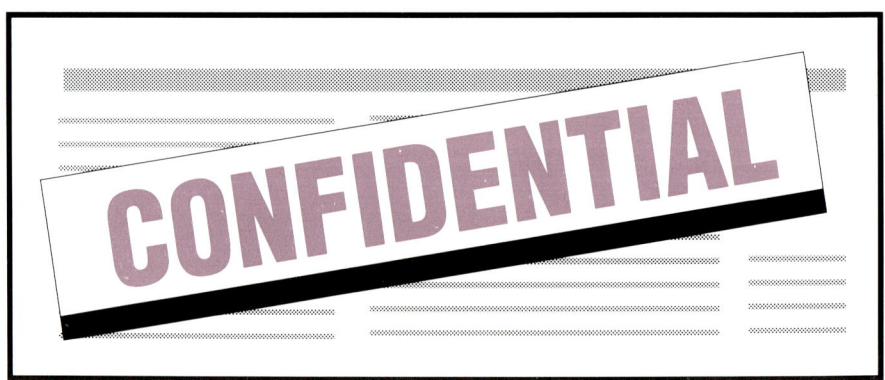

Figure 2.1

EXERCISE 2.1

● What is your employer's policy on confidentiality? If there is no formal policy, what expectations of you do your employers have (with regard to confidentiality)?

● If you work with children: Do you know where a copy of the child protection procedures are and what the obligations are?

● If you work with adults: Are there policies or procedures relating to the protection of adults which apply to you? Do you know what your obligations are?

Your task in this exercise is to ensure that you are able to answer the above questions. You may need to consult written documents of policies and procedures and/or spend some time with your line manager or a senior colleague in order to get the information you need.

Boundaries

A boundary is a dividing line or limit. Boundaries are therefore an important aspect of confidentiality - they raise the key question of: Where do you draw the line? This can be seen to apply in a number of ways. Let's consider each of these in turn.

Who should know?

Where do we draw the line between who should know and who should not? To answer this question, you will need to consider:

- The nature of the information given;
- the wishes of the person giving the information;
- your employer's policy on confidentiality and storage of information;
- legal requirements (see Appendix II);
- other requirements, for example, child protection procedures.

What needs to be recorded?

Obviously, not all information given by service users can or should be entered in written records. So, how do we decide what gets written down and what does not? There is no simple or straight forward answer to this question and so we shall look at it in more detail below.

When should confidentiality be over-ridden?

Confidentiality is a right and, as such, it can only be over-ridden in exceptional circumstances. The general principle will be discussed below under the heading of 'Rights and Choice'. However, as confidentiality is such a thorny issue, it is worth devoting some time to these issues here. The key word is that of protection, whether the protection of the individual concerned or the protection of others. A helpful way of understanding this is to regard information given in confidence as sacrosanct unless and until this comes into conflict with your duty to safeguard the health and well-being of those in your care, your colleagues and others, including the community at large. Examples of such conflict would be:

- *suicide risk* - This type of information must be passed on, even though this may create a moral dilemma for you if the person concerned asks you to keep the information to yourself;

● *risk to others* - This covers a wide range of possibilities and includes risk of infection or an intention to harm someone else;

● *protection procedures* - Child protection procedures have been in existence for many years but, increasingly, official procedures are now being set up in relation to other vulnerable groups at risk of abuse. It is essential that you are aware of your obligations under the appropriate procedures and that you abide by them.

If you should find yourself in a situation where such a conflict applies, it is important that you do not carry the responsibility for the problem on your own. Make sure you discuss the situation with your line manager or another senior colleague. If you do not, you could find yourself not only in a stressful dilemma but also, quite possibly, in a situation where you are being held partly responsible for a harmful outcome or even subject to a disciplinary charge.

Official records

It is, of course, common practice for social care organisations to keep official records, whether in manual files, on computer, or both. Such records have important implications for confidentiality in terms of:

1 What is kept on record and for how long;
2 Who has access to such records in normal circumstances;
3 Who else has access to the records in exceptional circumstances;
4 Whether the records are securely stored.

1 *What is kept on record and for how long will depend largely on the policy and established practices of your employers. It is therefore important that you make sure that you have a clear understanding of what is expected of you as far as written records are concerned. In particular, a very important question to ask is: What sort of things have to be put on record? Some types of information may have to be recorded even if you were asked to keep the information secret. The point to note here is that the information you receive is received on behalf of the organisation you work for.*

*That is, the information given belongs not to you
personally, but to your employing organisation.*

2   *To maintain confidentiality, we have to be clear about
who is allowed to have access to records. It is then the
responsibility of staff to ensure that unauthorised
persons do not have access to confidential information.
Care therefore needs to be taken to make sure that
records are not left lying around or allowed to get into
the hands of the wrong people.*

3   *At certain times, other people may have a right to see
the information kept on record. Examples of this
would be formal inquiries or investigations, or court
cases. Complaints and representation procedures may
well result in wider access to records by senior staff or
independant arbiters.*

4   *There is, of course, little point in trying to maintain
confidentiality if records are not securely kept. Are
written records kept under lock and key? Are computer
records protected from unauthorised access? These are
important and significant questions - as indeed, are the
key questions of: 'What part do I play in keeping
confidential records secure? 'and' What are my
responsibilities in safeguarding confidentiality?'*

How we deal with records in particular and confidentiality in
general will depend, to a large extent, on the policies and
expectations of our employers. These, in turn, will largely depend
on legal requirements and guidelines. Space does not permit a
detailed exploration of the legal framework of confidentiality but a
summary of the main points of law appears as Appendix 2.

Guidelines for good practice

As we have seen, confidentiality is a complex subject and one
which can cause a number of problems if it is not handled carefully
and sensitively. This pack cannot ensure that you do not encounter
any of these problems but the guidance we give here can, we
hope, help you to minimise the chances of things going wrong. We
therefore offer the following guidelines as helpful suggestions for
dealing with the thorny issues of confidentiality.

EXERCISE 2.2

The object of this exercise is to make sure that you are clear about what is expected of you in terms of record-keeping. As with Exercise 2.1. you should consult official policy documents and/or use your line manager or colleagues as a source of information and advice. The questions you need to address are:

1   Does your employer have a formal policy on record-keeping? If so, what are your obligations? If no formal policy exists, what does your employer expect of you?

2   Who has access to the records? Who else may have access to the records in certain circumstances? Do service users have access to their records? What restrictions apply?

3   Are records securely kept? How do you prevent unauthorised persons from having access?

4   If you have any doubts, conflicts or dilemmas in relation to record keeping, where do you go for advice? Who has managerial responsibility for records?

1   *Be clear about your responsibilities*   As we have noted, confidentiality is a complex and thorny matter and so it is not too difficult to become confused and lose track of the issues. When this happens, it is then quite easy for confidentiality to be breached inadvertently. Confidential information can so easily 'slip out' inappropriately with potentially disastrous results. It is therefore imperative that you are clear about your responsibilities with regard to confidentiality, that you take them seriously and that you are vigilant.

2   *Inform service users of where they stand*   As confidentiality is not an absolute right, you will need to make sure that service users (and others who may give you information in confidence) are clear about:

- Where and how information will be stored;
- Who will have access to it;
- In what circumstances confidentiality will be over-ridden and with what consequences;
- What rights the individual has with regard to obtaining access to the information stored.

It is helpful if these matters can be clarified sooner, rather than later. If not, you run the risk of creating a very difficult situation in which people feel you have misled them or hidden things from them. Clearly, this makes working on the basis of trust a very difficult undertaking.

3   *Obtain proof of identity when necessary*   It is possible for confidential information to 'fall into the wrong hands' if we are lax in passing on information. For example, if we do not check the identity of people requesting information, we may be guilty of passing on that information to people who have no right to it. Social care staff are under an obligation to maintain confidentiality and so it is important to seek proof of identity whenever there is any doubt. If, for example, someone makes a telephone enquiry, it may be necessary to ask for his or her telephone number and ring back, having first checked that it is a bonafide number for the agency concerned.

4   *Don't be afraid to ask for help*   Dealing with the potential conflicts and dilemmas of confidentiality is a

demanding task and one that can give rise to a lot of worry and pressure. This being the case, it is important that you know where to get advice and support. But, just knowing where to get help is not enough - you've got to actually use that help when you need to. Asking for help is not a sign of weakness. Rather, it is a sign of professional commitment to working together to provide the best care for your service users.

5 *Try to create an atmosphere of trust* The importance of maintaining confidentiality can become just a hollow phrase if there is no atmosphere of trust in which people feel able to talk about personal and private matters, to discuss their worries and concerns. Without this atmosphere of trust, people can feel lonely, isolated and unsupported. In this way, extra barriers and tensions are created which, in turn, create additional pressures and problems for service users and staff alike. Of course, generating an atmosphere of trust is no easy or straightforward matter. But, one thing which can make a significant contribution is, ironically maintaining confidentiality. Trust and confidentiality reinforce each other. Trying to achieve one without the other is likely to prove an extremely difficult, if not impossible, task.

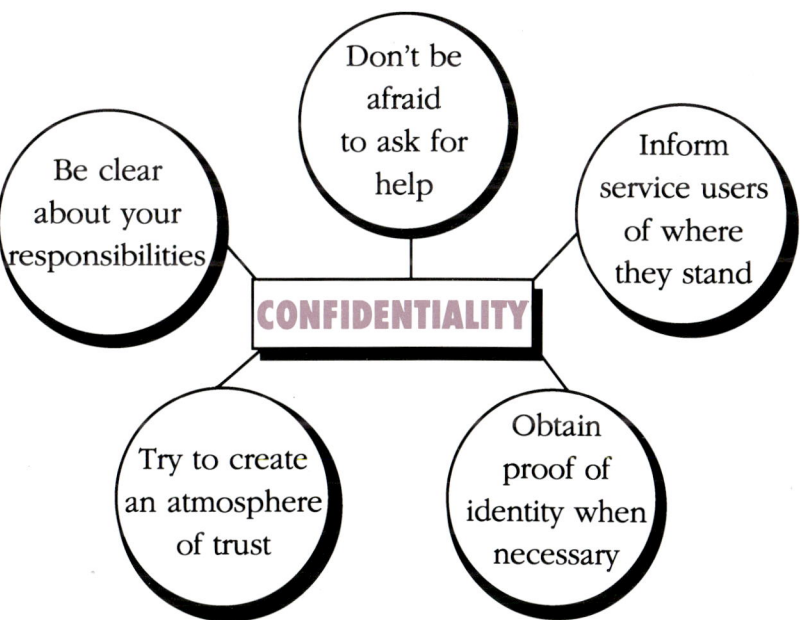

Figure 2.2

Conclusion

Working in social care often means dealing with vulnerable people at a personal level. This makes your job a very important and responsible one - and one that can easily go sadly wrong if we are not careful. Confidentiality is therefore very significant in this respect. If it is handled well, it plays an important part in the provision of high quality social care. But, if it is not handled well, it can cause major problems, leaving people feeling betrayed, unsupported and under-valued. We very much hope that this pack can help you to make sure, as far as possible, that the outcomes you achieve are positive ones.

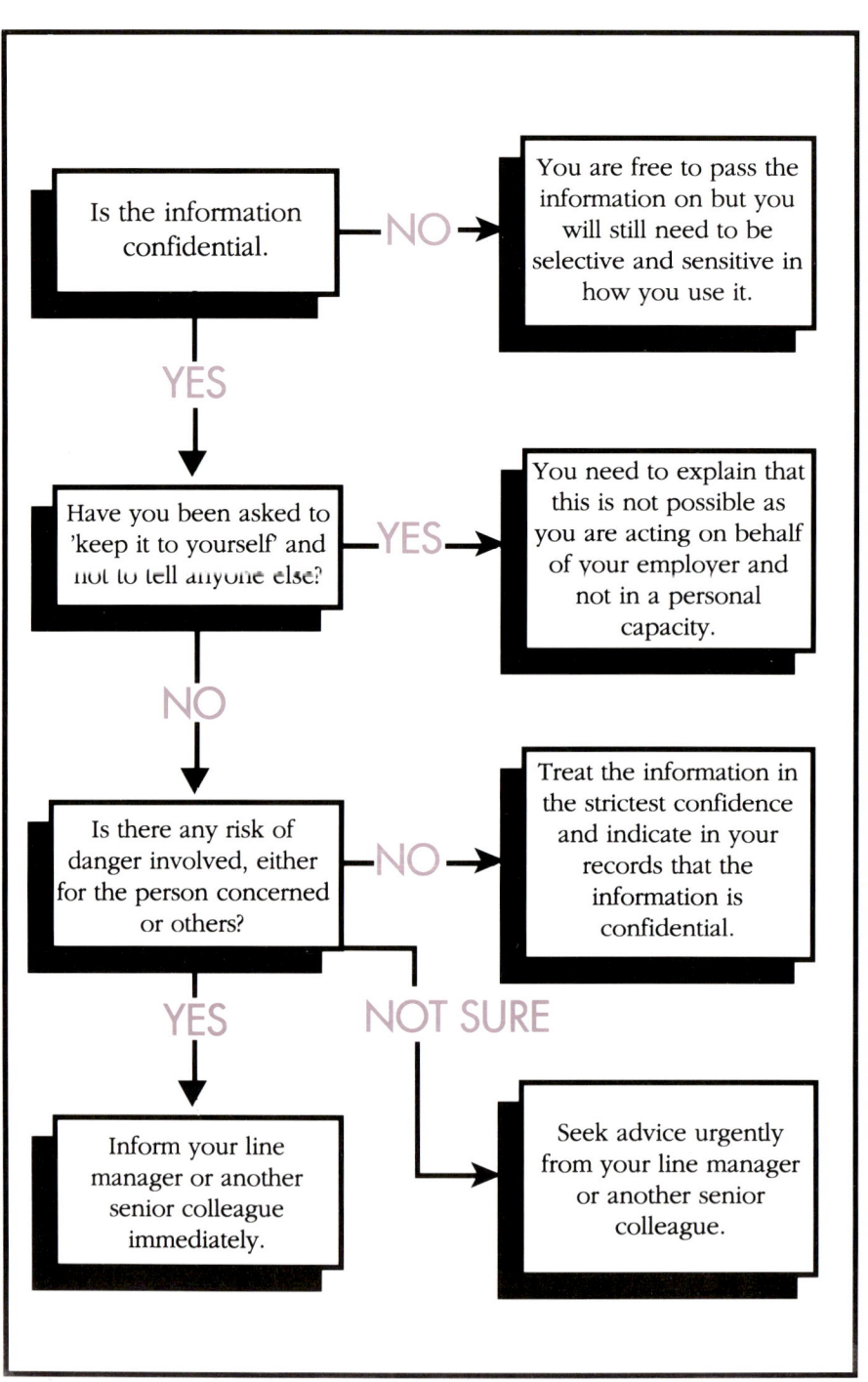

Figure 2.3

44

NOTES

NOTES

NOTES

NOTES

3

Rights and Choice

ELEMENT O.c
Promote and support individual rights and choice within service delivery

Why are rights and choice important?

Rights and choice are both important aspects of human dignity and are therefore an essential part of the value base of social care. People in need of social care are, first and foremost, citizens and, as such, have basic rights. In this part of the pack we shall look in more detail at what these rights are and how these can be safeguarded. Also, we need to be clear about the circumstances in which an individual's rights can be over-ruled, either for his or her own good or for the protection of others. Choice is also an important part of citizenship, an essential part of living a satisfying and fulfilling life. Choice is about having some degree of control over one's life. The absence of choice is therefore both oppressive and, as we shall see, a significant source of stress and distress.

What are rights?

The Webster's Third New International Dictionary defines a right as: 'something to which one has a just claim... the power or privilege to which one is justly entitled', a definition which seems to hinge on two key concepts - justice, or fairness, and entitlement. Fairness is, of course, a central value in social work and social care and reflects the importance, discussed in Part 1 of this pack, of an approach based on equality of opportunity. Entitlement implies that a right is not a matter of discretion, it is not something that can be withheld without good reason. Clearly then, rights are an important part of the value base of working with people in need of social care. Understanding people's rights, and working sensitively and effectively with them, is therefore a fundamental aspect of good practice. Perhaps the best way to understand rights is to look at a range of examples and consider, briefly at least, some of the implications for practice. This is precisely what we shall do in the next section.

Service users have a right to...

Equality of treatment. As we made clear in Part 1 of the pack, equality is a primary value in social care. It is, of course, also a fundamental right and one we would do well not to ignore. It is clearly a matter of good practice to ensure that people are not unfairly treated on the basis of gender, colour, ethnic group, age, disability, sexual orientation or any other such factors. It is therefore vitally important that staff are sensitive to the potential for discrimination and unfair treatment.

Privacy   In group care settings there is sometimes a problem over privacy. There can be difficulties in trying to give people the space to be on their own when they feel the need to. However, we should be careful to ensure that we do not become defeatist about this and assume that privacy is not possible. It is important that a person's wish for privacy is respected as the absence of privacy can lead to considerable tension, distress and even depression. A common mistake as far as privacy is concerned is to assume that people who enjoy the company of others do not want or need privacy. The important point here is that people should be given the choice - an issue to which we shall return below. Privacy is particularly important with regard to personal matters such as bathing, toileting and so on. This can be a difficult issue for people whose personal care needs are quite extensive and who may need direct assistance in such matters. In such cases, the need for staff to handle the situation with great sensitivity and dignity is paramount.

Information and consultation   Social care is a service we provide for those people who need it. As such, it is not something that we do *to* people, but rather *with* them. It is therefore important that service users are fully involved in planning, both on a day to day basis and in the longer term. For this to be effective it is necessary for full consultation to take place at every stage and for no information to be withheld. Information and consultation are essential parts of empowerment - key aspects of the process of helping people gain as much control as possible over their lives and circumstances. It is therefore important that social care practice contributes positively to this process by ensuring appropriate consultation and information, as a failure to do so can be seen as a significant denial of a basic right in social care.

Confidentiality   Just as there is a right to receive information, so too is there a right for information about, or from, service users to be treated in confidence, subject to the constraints already discussed in Part 2 of this pack.

Individuality and identity   Each service user has a right to be treated as a unique individual and a person in their own right. The implications of this form the subject matter of the next part of the pack and so we shall not comment further at this stage.

Respect and self-respect Respect is a quality that is rather intangible but none the less important and worthy of attention. Having respect for people involves:

- being prepared to listen;
- not trying to impose your own view;
- going at their pace;
- taking account of their feelings and needs;
- not being condescending or over-bearing;
- not seeing yourself as being in any way superior.

Good practice in social care must therefore not only recognise these points but also ensure that they are adhered to, that is, based in reality rather than just paid lip service. Self-respect is an extension of this and is closely related to self-esteem, the value we place upon ourselves. Simply put, self-respect and therefore self-esteem, will be seriously hampered by an absence of respect on the part of others.

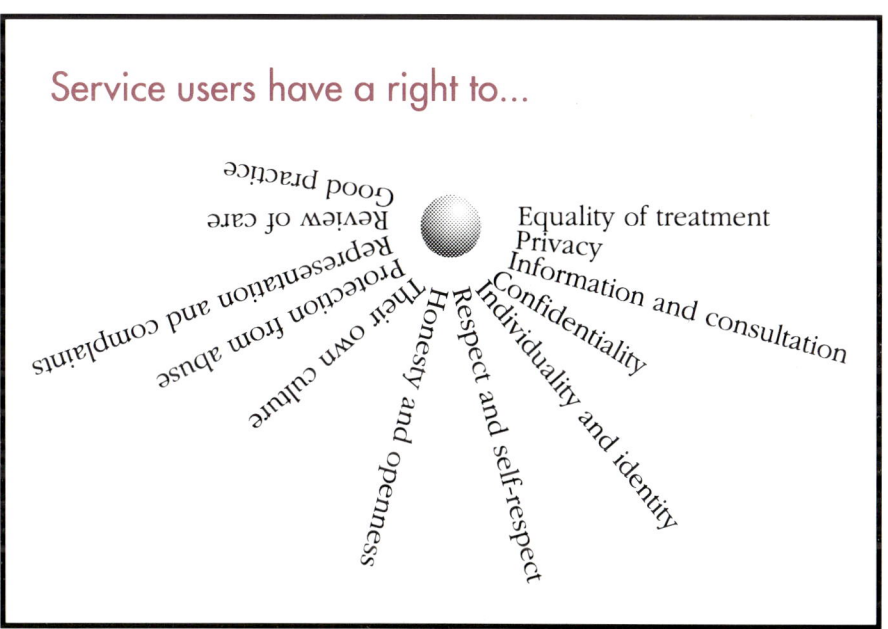

Service users have a right to...

Good practice
Review of care
Representation
Protection from abuse
Their own culture
Honesty and openness
Respect and self-respect
Individuality and identity
Confidentiality
Information and consultation
Privacy
Equality of treatment
Representation and complaints

Figure 3.1

Honesty and openess This follows on from the previous point. We can hardly claim to be dealing with people in a respectful way if we are less than honest or if we keep secrets. For service users to feel secure and settled there must be an atmosphere of mutual trust. Such an atmosphere is, of course, not possible unless complete honesty is established as the norm. Even the slightest example of dishonesty can destroy months or even years of building up trust and mutual respect.

Their own culture Cultural customs, practices, expectations and beliefs play a major part in our lives. For these to be over-ridden,

EXERCISE 3.1

Think about the service users you are currently working with.
What cultural backgrounds are represented (for example,
religions or languages? In what ways do you (and your
colleagues) take account of different cultural backgrounds?
Does your employing organisation have a policy on race/
ethnictary/culture? If so, do you know what its implications are
for you?

These are important questions. Spend some time thinking about
them, discuss them with your colleagues and use the space
below to make some notes.

ignored, marginalised, discredited or ridiculed is clearly a form of oppression and therefore, by definition, bad practice. Good practice therefore needs to be 'ethnically-sensitive', aware of, and responsive to, different cultural values and needs. As mentioned in Part 1, this is an important part of anti-discriminatory practice. However, we should note that this is not simply a matter of differences between black and white. Within both black and white communities there is a considerable diversity of cultures in terms of:

- language;
- religion;
- national or regional identity.

Such differences can manifest themselves in a variety of ways (for example diet) and can have major implications for social care practice. If our attempts to provide care are not to prove oppressive, we must ensure that we take full account of the cultural background of the people we work with.

Protection from abuse Abuse is, by definition, something to be avoided, something from which we all need to be protected as far as possible. In general, the more vulnerable a person is, the greater the risk of abuse. As people in need of social care are so often vulnerable in some way, they tend to be more prone to abuse than others (consider, for example, both child abuse and the abuse of older people - 'elder abuse'). In order to protect people from abuse, we need to:

- be sensitive to the possibility of abuse and recognise the danger signs;
- be aware of policies and procedures relating to abuse and the responsibilities these place on us;
- share any concerns we may have with our line manager or senior colleague;
- ensure that our own actions and attitudes are in no way abusive.

The right to protection from abuse is an extremely important right for, without this right, so many other rights lose all meaning.

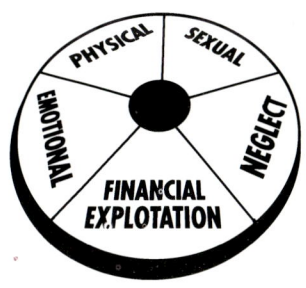

Figure 3.2
Types of abuse

Representation and complaints Service users have a right to make complaints where necessary and to be represented. This is important for two reasons:

1 Knowing that access to a helpful complaints procedure is available gives service users a sense of security, a safety-net which can reassure them that they will be listened to if there is anything they are unhappy about.

2 Similarly, from the staff's point of view, the complaints procedure can act as a spur to good practice by:

- identifying possible areas of bad practice and thus providing learning opportunities;
- clearing up possible misunderstandings or tensions between staff and service users;
- emphasising the need for high quality care.

It is important, therefore, that the complaints procedure is not seen in a negative light as a threat or a problem. It has a very positive and constructive role to play in ensuring that the care provided is of the highest quality possible within the resources available.

Review of care Once care arrangements are established, the planning task is, of course, not complete. These arrangements will need to be reviewed to take account of changing circumstances or new information gained. Satisfactory care arrangements can easily become very unsatisfactory if the situation is not reviewed on a regular basis.

Good practice In a sense, this is the sum of all the other rights. Without good practice service users can be harmed rather than helped, oppressed rather than empowered. Having a need for care means being dependent, to a certain extent, on staff. This makes service users very vulnerable to the negative effects of bad practice. Rights are, of course, closely linked with duties. As we have seen, service users have a number of important rights, and so this means that service providers, that is, staff, have certain duties. Perhaps the most important of these duties, and certainly the most central one, is the duty to avoid bad practice wherever possible, the duty to ensure that the standards of care provided are the best possible within the resources available.

EXERCISE 3.2

Does your employing organisation have a Representation and Complaints procedure? If so, what are your obligations under this procedure? (What do you need to know and what do you need to do?).

If there is no official procedure, what do your employers expect of you in this respect? Are you clear what your role is and how you should proceed if a complaint needs to be made? Use the space below to make some notes.

The significance of choice

The notion of choice implies two sets of issues, both of which have a major bearing on social care:

1 *Options* There needs to be a range of options available for choice to have any real meaning. Do the people you work with have real choices? Do you play a part in increasing these options and do you make sure people know what options are available?

2 *The opportunity to choose* Clearly, it is no good having options available if people are not given the opportunity to choose, if decisions are made for them or, if no consultation takes place. It is not enough to have options available in theory - there must be genuine choice in practice.

It must be remembered that choice is not a luxury but, rather, an essential element of good quality care. We cannot expect people to have dignity and self-respect and to feel happy and settled unless they have as much control over their lives as possible.

When should rights and choice be over-ridden?

This is a difficult but, none the less, important question and one that we have already encountered in relation to confidentiality. The key word here is risk and relates to the sort of situation in which exercising a particular right or choice may place someone in danger. This applies in two ways:

1 *Danger to others* The risk factors are likely to vary across the different client groups but the common theme is that certain restrictions on a person's rights or choice may be necessary in order to safeguard others (for example, a prohibition on smoking in certain areas).

2 *Danger to oneself* This is less clear-cut and places us in something of a moral dilemma. Certain actions can place people at risk of injury or even death but do we have the right to protect people from their own actions even if this goes against their wishes? In general terms, the answer is 'no', although we do have a duty to dissuade people from harmful actions.

It is clearly the second aspect, danger to oneself, that is more complex and more difficult to deal with. A helpful concept in trying to wrestle with these issues is that of responsibility. It is our responsibility to try to discourage or dissuade people from taking steps that can, or will lead to self-harm. However, we are not responsible for the consequences if they decide to go ahead regardless of our discouragement or disapproval, except in the case of any of the following three sets of circumstances applying:

1 *The self-harm would also be a danger to others*
Sometimes we can concentrate so much on the element of self-harm that we lose track of the possibility of harm to others.

2 *The person concerned is a child*   Here it is necessary to act in *loco parentis* and to protect the child from harm.

3 *The person concerned is mentally disordered or has severe learning difficulties*   In such situations, the Mental Health Act 1983 will apply and you will need to get specialist help.

Any situation which involves denying some one their rights or choice is a very serious one which should not be taken lightly. It is advisable that, wherever you encounter such a situation - actually or potentially - you seek the advice of your line manager or a senior colleague.

Conclusion

In studying the value base of social care, rights and choice are bound to play a significant part. As we have seen, it is both a complex and vitally important area, a key aspect of good practice which places a range of demands on staff. Earlier, under the heading of 'service users have a right to... Good practice', the point was made that a set of rights implies a set of duties. This section of the pack has, we hope, helped you to form a picture of what those duties are and how you might tackle them. We hope it has also shown you how important these matters are and has encouraged you to learn more about them and develop your skills further.

NOTES

Individuality and Identity

ELEMENT O.d
Acknowledge individuals' personal beliefs and identity

Why are individuality and identity important?

As with rights and choice, individuality and identity are important aspects of human dignity. If people feel they are not being treated as individuals but simply as part of a wider group, it is likely that they will feel that their needs are not being recognised and that they are not being valued as a person in their own right. Such an experience can be a profoundly alienating and dehumanising one and, therefore, very oppressive. People in need of social care may well have much in common, but we should not allow this to distract us from the fact that each one is a unique individual with a specific identity.

What are individuality and identity?

In some ways, all people are the same. For example, we all need to eat, drink, breathe and so on. In some ways, some people are the same and some are different. For example, in terms of age, gender, culture and other social group membership, we will have much in common with certain groups of people but will be very different from others. In some ways, all people are unique, with their own personal beliefs, feelings and needs. It is at this third level that individuality and identity are very much to the fore. Identity is, of course, a short-hand term for who we are, the sense of self that we have. This can be divided into two main elements - self-image and self-esteem:

Self-image describes the view we have of ourselves, the image on which we base our thoughts, feelings and actions. For example, it is recognised that people suffering from anorexia nervosa tend to have an image of themselves as fat even though they are, in reality, quite thin.

Self-esteem refers to the value we place on ourselves, how highly we think of ourselves. High self-esteem is associated with confidence and a positive attitude, whilst low self-esteem is associated with feelings of worthlessness, low motivation and, in extreme cases, depression.

Both these concepts, self-image and self-esteem, are important in providing high quality social care in so far as good practice involves making sure we contribute, as far as possible, to a positive self-image and high self-esteem.

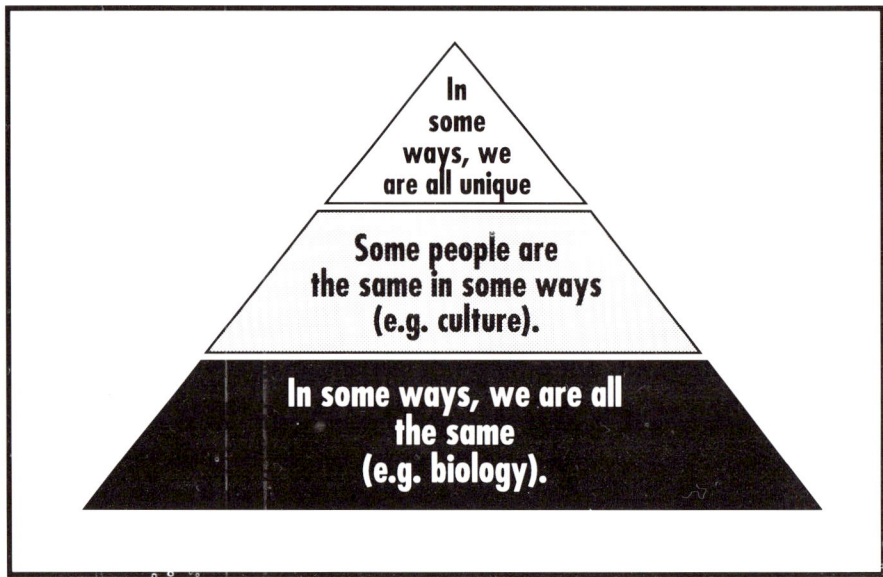

*Figure 4.1
The uniqueness
of the individual*

Personal beliefs

A person's beliefs and values are an important part of his or her sense of identity and are a key part of:

- the past - previous life experiences and socialisation;
- the present - our beliefs have a significant influence on our actions and attitudes;
- the future - our wishes, aspirations and plans.

What we have to bear in mind, therefore, is that personal beliefs are very significant for the individual. Consequently, to dismiss, disregard or invalidate a person's beliefs is to dismiss, disregard or invalidate the person. Where such beliefs are a reflection of a person's religion or culture, then that religion or culture can be under attack too. It is to be hoped that social care staff would not act in such a way intentionally, although such problems do arise at certain times. However, what is much more likely to happen than a deliberate attack on someone's beliefs or culture is to cause offence unintentionally. The underlying problem is therefore more likely to be one of insensitivity or lack of awareness than one of malice. Consequently, an important aspect of good practice in terms of individualism and identity is to develop a sensitivity to matters of culture, religion and language - to develop what was called in Part 1, ethnically-sensitive practice. It is also important to recognise that there can be a conflict between your own beliefs and those of the people you work with. Sometimes, this is open and it is easy to see the differences. However, at other times, the differences can be more hidden and implicit - more difficult to spot but, none the less, powerful in their influence and their potential for conflict. An example of the latter would be differences based on class background. Sometimes, people from different backgrounds feel uncomfortable with each other but cannot quite put their finger on what the problem is. When such situations arise, it is important to recognise what is happening so that tensions between you do not increase and lead to a problematic situation. It is a good idea to try to work out just what the differences are between you so that you can try to find common ground and establish a good working relationship. In order to do this you may need to talk over the situation with your line manager or someone else you trust, someone who can take a more objective view of the situation.

Our beliefs and values are, in a sense, the spectacles through which we view the world. As such, they have a significant impact on our day to day lives in terms of:

- our tastes and preferences;
- what motivates us;
- what we find offensive;
- what makes us feel comfortable or uncomfortable;
- our hopes and fears.

For this reason, it is essential, from the point of view of good social care practice, to understand what people's beliefs and values are and, as far as possible, to respect them.

Knowing and assuming

A lot of the time we get these two mixed up - we act as if we know something when, in fact, we are making an assumption. Of course, it would be impossible to check everything out and make sure of our facts. It is inevitable that we will have to rely on assumptions to a certain extent. However, what tends to be very problematic is when we do not appreciate the difference between knowing and assuming. This is particularly the case in terms of stereotypes. Stereotypes are fixed and rigid views of certain people or groups of people which we are unlikely to change, even in the face of strong evidence to the contrary. A stereotype is therefore a form of prejudice - a pre-judgement or false generalisation that distorts our perception of the person or the group of people:

EXERCISE 4.1

Who are you? To understand the importance of other people's individuality and identity, it is helpful to get a picture of your own sense of self. Use the grid below to help you with this.

How would you describe yourself? What key words would you use?

Who are the important people in your life?

What values and beliefs do you hold dear?

What activities (hobbies or work, for example) are particularly important to you?

What have you achieved that you feel proud of?

And finally, how would you feel if any of the above were threatened, disregarded or dismissed by someone that you have to rely upon?

The concept of stereotyping is a particularly important one in relation to discrimination and oppression. Dominance, inequality and injustice are often maintained by reference to stereotypes, for example, of black people, of women, of old or disabled people. Stereotypes are therefore powerful tools of ideology and are thus significant obstacles to the development of anti-discriminatory practice. (Thompson, 1993, p. 27)

What this shows is that there is a danger of being too rigid or dogmatic in our beliefs. It is important that we are able to be flexible and responsive, rather than allow ourselves to get stuck in the tramlines of stereotypical thinking. It is essential that we get to know the individual, rather than simply make assumptions about him or her, otherwise there is a danger that we are making a false generalisation - an experience which could be profoundly alienating or oppressive for the service user concerned. A particularly problematic aspect of this is when service users become stereotyped as a group in their own right - 'That's typical of the people here'. This reflects the very harmful process of institutionalisation in which individualism and personal identity are swallowed up in the interests of simplifying the situation so that it is easier for staff to deal with. You need to be very wary of this process as it is a very destructive one. Individuals become treated just as examples of 'the sort of people we have here' rather than individuals in their own right. Often, the language used can reflect or reinforce this process of 'de-individualisation'. For example, terms like 'the elderly' or 'the handicapped' are very impersonal and have derogatory overtones. Terms like 'older people' or 'people with a disability' are far less problematic and are therefore very much to be preferred.

Guidelines for good practice

Getting to grips with the complex issues of individualism and identity can be quite tricky and demanding. To help you with this task, the remainder of this part of the pack is devoted to a number of guidelines for good practice - practical pointers to help you develop your skills and confidence in this area. It is to be hoped that these guidelines will help you, and encourage you, to think further about the issues, rather than simply provide you with a set of 'dos' and 'don'ts' that you follow unthinkingly.

EXERCISE 4.2

This is an exercise about stereotypes and assumptions. First of all, let's consider you as a stereotype. What would the stereotype of a social care worker be (in your particular area practice)? Consult with your colleagues if need be and make some notes in the space below

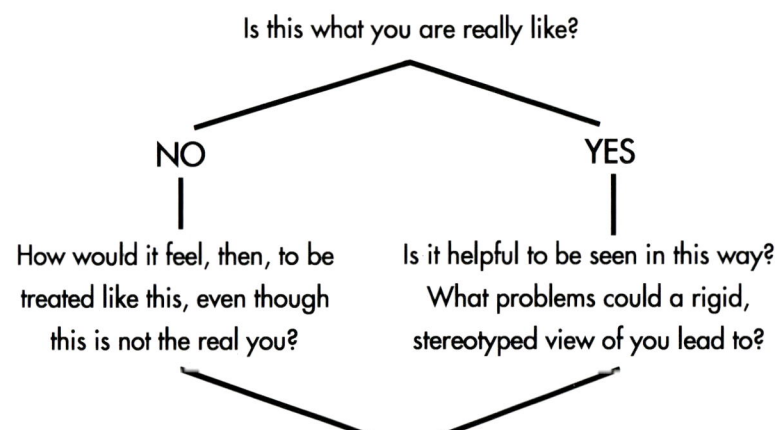

Is this what you are really like?

NO   YES

How would it feel, then, to be   Is it helpful to be seen in this way?
treated like this, even though   What problems could a rigid,
this is not the real you?   stereotyped view of you lead to?

What are the implications for practice? What should you do to prevent stereotypes from becoming a barrier to good social care? Make some notes in the space below (consult with colleagues if you wish).

1 Respect people's rights

As we saw in Part 3 of this pack, rights and choice play an important part in social care. We can now further recognise that undermining a person's rights also amounts to undermining his or her individuality by devaluing the person and thereby attacking his or her self-esteem.

2 Be sensitive to cultural issues

As we have seen, a person's cultural background is a central part of his or her identity or sense of self. We must therefore make sure that we take account of such matters by developing our knowledge, awareness and understanding of different cultural beliefs, values, practices and needs.

3 Adopt an anti-racist approach

Whilst it is clearly important to develop an ethnically-sensitive approach, this on its own is not enough. We also have to recognise that society devalues certain cultures and sees them as inferior. This being the case, many service users will have experienced racism, and the hostility and rejection this entails. This has three sets of implications:

- these issues need to be taken into account in terms of your assessment of people's needs;
- you need to make sure your own actions and attitudes do not unwittingly reinforce such racism;
- you need to challenge and undermine racism whenever you encounter it.

4 Acknowledge the individual as a person

Sometimes, in dealing with a lot of people, and with a lot of tasks to complete, we can slip into bad habits of forgetting to treat people as individuals. When this happens, social care becomes nothing more than meeting basic needs and loses track of higher goals of quality of life and the need to feel valued as a person in your own right. Being busy explains why this often gets forgotten but, of course, it does not excuse it.

5 Be prepared to listen

If we work on the basis of stereotypes and assumptions, we do not need to listen as we already 'know' the answer. However, if we are to avoid this type of practice, we need to make sure that we are really listening to what people are trying to say to us. This is a point which will be discussed in more detail in the next part of the pack.

6 Address people appropriately

Our names, and how we are addressed by people, are also important parts of our sense of identity. In order to respect this we must check how people wish to be addressed. For example, in dealing with adults, beware of assuming that using first names will be interpreted as a sign of friendship. Many people were brought up to see this a sign of a lack of respect and may prefer the use of formal titles (e.g. Mr. or Mrs.) until they get to know you. It does not hurt to ask people how they would prefer to be addressed - but it can hurt to be addressed inappropriately. Similarly, in working with children or adults, beware of using nicknames without first checking that this is acceptable to the person concerned. Do not assume that the nickname is welcomed by the service user (or that you have yet earned the right to use that nickname if it is a sign of affection or friendship).

7 Seek guidance where necessary

As we acknowledged before, these are complex matters so do not be afraid to ask your colleagues or your line manager for guidance. It is also helpful to get the views of others on these matters as they are very personal and you can find it difficult to see them objectively if you do not have the benefit of other people's perspectives. Seeking guidance from others is an important part of learning.

8 Know yourself

This is a bit of a cliché and is certainly easier said than done. However, self-awareness - knowing about your own individuality and identity - is certainly a very helpful and constructive step on the path towards appreciating the importance of these matters for the people you work with. It is to be hoped that Exercise 4.1 has helped you to begin this process and that you will continue with it.

Conclusion

One of the traditional criticisms of social care, especially residential care, is that service users lose their dignity and self-respect because they lose their independence and their ability to control their own lives. Certainly this is a valid criticism of bad practice in social care. It would be extremely unfair, though, to 'tar all social care with the same brush'. Good practice in social care, based on promoting individuality and identity, clearly does not deserve this criticism as such an approach can be seen to empower people, to give them as much control as possible over their lives, to make a positive contribution to self-esteem and to discourage dependency as far as possible.

In view of this, the challenge to promote individuality and identity within social care is a major one but, none the less, a vital one.

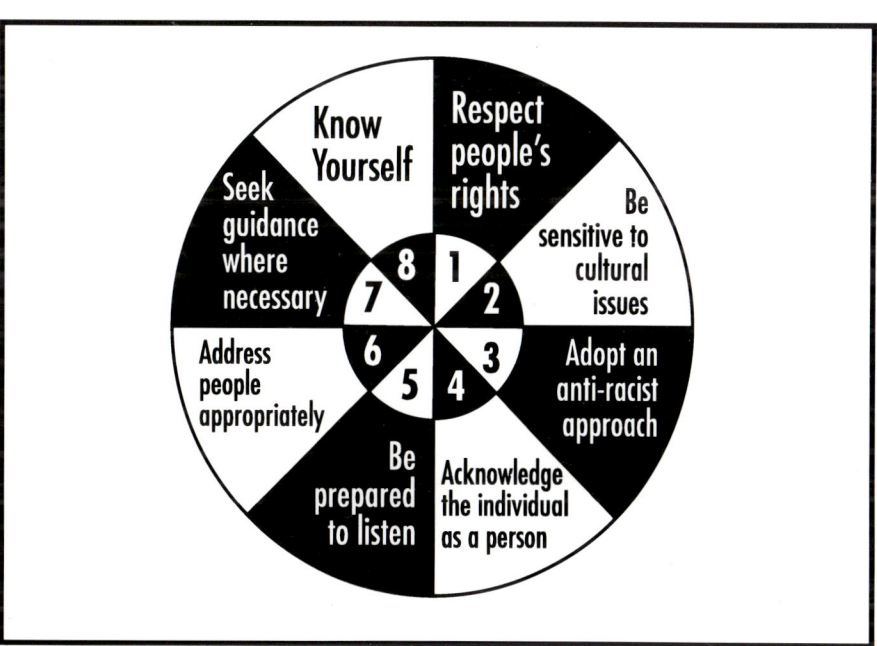

Figure 4.2
Guidelines
for good
practice

NOTES

NOTES

72

5

Communication Skills

ELEMENT O.e
Support individuals through effective communication

Why are communication skills important?

Communication is not only a fundamental part of social care but also a basic part of social life itself. Whatever we are communicating - or trying to communicate - the implications of getting it wrong can be of major proportions. Social care is about dealing with people and that necessarily involves communication. The quality of our interactions with others is therefore dependent, to a large extent, on our ability to communicate effectively and appropriately. Consequently, the skills involved in communication, the barriers to good communication, and possible strategies for removing such barriers are all very significant in terms of the promotion and maintenance of good social care practice.

What are communication skills?

Communication involves the transmission of information. This can be in a variety of ways - written, verbal and non-verbal. The people involved in communicating can either help or hinder the transmission of information. This is where skills have an important part to play - communication skills can help to make sure that what we do helps rather than hinders. These skills include:

- expressing yourself clearly;
- active listening;
- sensitivity to body language;
- recognising barriers to communication.

The remainder of this part of the pack examines these and other skills under three separate headings - verbal, non-verbal and written. By considering each of these three areas, it is to be hoped that you will be able to develop a greater awareness of the intricacies of communication and a greater confidence in dealing with them.

Speaking and listening - verbal skills

Some people find it very easy to communicate even in difficult circumstances, but most of us have to work at it, to develop the skills and sensitivity necessary. Much of this will come from experience but we can, none the less, help the process along by improving our understanding of what makes for good communication - and what gets in the way. Perhaps one of the most important aspects of verbal communication is putting people at their ease. If the person(s) you are talking to do not feel at ease, it is quite possible that they will not be taking on board what you are saying or it may be distorted. Verbal communication is therefore not just about the words we use but also about a range of other factors. It is useful, in trying to maximise the effectiveness of communication, to address the following issues:

● Is this the right time and place? For example, confidential matters should not be discussed in front of others;

● Have you set the right tone? For example, is it clear to the person(s) you are speaking to whether this is to be a 'chat' or more formal discussion?

● Are you being clear and unambiguous? For example, are you sure what you are saying is not likely to be misinterpreted?

● Do you listen? This is a key question and one which merits closer attention.

Active listening

Listening is more than just hearing - it means actually taking on board what is being said to you and showing that you understand. It means engaging with someone, and not simply being present when they are speaking. The term 'active listening' is used to describe the process whereby you not only listen effectively but also communicate that you are doing so. This process involves:

● Thinking carefully about what is being said to you without jumping to conclusions or relying on pre-conceived notions;

● Acknowledging feelings; for example, if someone is feeling angry, it can help if you acknowledge this;

● Actively showing that you are listening (eye contact, nodding, smiling and so on);

EXERCISE 5.1

This is an exercise in active listening and is in two parts. First, choose a person you think of as a good listener. What is it that makes him or her a good listener. Think carefully about this and make some notes in the space below. If you feel it is appropriate, it may also be helpful to talk to the person concerned and find out what he or she thinks is important in effective listening.

The second part involves you trying to put this learning into practice.
Practise your skills in active listening by trying to listen as attentively as possible to someone, bearing in mind what you learned from the first part of this exercise.
Try not to think of this as an exercise to be done just once. It is something that you can keep doing from time to time and thereby build up on your listening skills.

● Not interrupting; interrupting people can give the impression that you feel that what you have to say is more important than what they have to say;

● Reflect back what has been said; you have to do this selectively as it gets tedious if you reflect back everything that is said. However, for some things - particularly very important matters - it is useful to relay back what you have heard to check that it has been understood.

Active listening is a positive and supportive way of interacting with people and so the skills are well worth developing. Exercise 5.1 is designed to help you with this.

Discriminatory	*Anti-Discriminatory*
man, mankind	people, humankind
to man	to staff, to cover
chairman,	chair, chairperson
a black day,	a bad day, a terrible day
to black	to boycott
black (in the sense of dirty)	dirty, grubby
the disabled,	disabled people,
the handicapped,	people with disabilities
the mentally	people with learning
handicapped,	difficulties/disabilities
the elderly.	older people, elders

This is not an extensive list but should be enough to give you a picture of the types of language that are problematic. The subject of discriminatory language is a complex one but, as a general rule, you should avoid terms that

● **exclude** — `every man for himself';

● **depersonalise** — `the elderly';

● **stigmatise** — `blackleg'.

*Figure 5.1
Discriminatory
Language*

Making yourself clear

One of the most significant barriers to effective communication is a lack of clarity. The following guidelines are intended to help you in this respect:

1 *Don't be vague*   Try to be as precise and explicit as you can. For example, do not say 'I'll be with you in a few minutes' when what you really mean is half or three quarters of an hour.

2 *Don't be ambiguous*   Try to avoid saying things that could be misinterpreted. For example, in 'Peter's social worker says he is pleased with the outcome' who is pleased, Peter or his social worker?

3 *Avoid slang and colloquialisms*   Slang is often local and so people from other areas, or from different cultures, may not understand certain words or phrases that you use. Slang is also often 'generational' in so far as people of a different age group may not use or understand certain terms.

4 *Articulate carefully*   This means, do not mumble; speak loudly enough (without shouting); do not speak too fast and do not 'block' speech (for example, by putting your hand over your mouth).

5 *Think first*   Sometimes people cannot express things clearly because they haven't got it clear in their minds what they are trying to say. In other words, if you're not sure what you are trying to say, do not be surprised when you fail to get your message across.

These are of course, not the only aspects of good verbal communication but they are a good starting point for you to begin developing your skills and knowledge.

Sensitivity

Another barrier to effective communication is a lack of sensitivity. There are three main ways in which this can apply:

1 *Special needs*   Sometimes, not enough account is taken of special communication needs, such as hearing or speech difficulties. If you deal with service users who have special needs as far as communication is concerned, it is important that you and your colleagues are sensitive to this and learn how best to deal with this situation.

2 *Personal background*   A person's religious, cultural and linguistic background are likely to have significant implications for communication. For example, if English is not a person's first language, it may be necessary to use an interpreter. Similarly, there may be cultural or religious matters that you need to take account of.

3 *Discrimination and oppression.*   A number of words and phrases need to be avoided as they can be seen to reinforce certain forms of discrimination and oppression or they are offensive to certain groups. Figure 5.1 lists many of the terms that are to be avoided and suggests some acceptable alternatives.

Putting it in writing

Keeping written records and writing reports can be a source of anxiety for social care staff. It would be sad indeed if this anxiety were allowed to act as a barrier to good practice. Consequently, the following guidelines are offered to help alleviate any such anxiety and clear up possible confusions.

1 *Plan in advance*   Sometimes, written work is of a poor standard largely because little or no forethought went into it. It is advisable to think carefully about what you want to say before you put pen to paper. That way, it makes it a lot easier to express yourself clearly and effectively.

2 *Make it relevant*   It is unrealistic to write everything down and so we have to make decisions about what is relevant and what is not. This is no easy matter but one which comes more easily with experience and skill development. One helpful guideline though, is to focus on the purpose of what you are writing. Thinking about why you are writing something will give you some clues as to what to include and what to leave out.

3 *Make a good impression*   Some people see grammar, spelling and punctuation as trivial and unimportant. However, such matters are important for two reasons. First, errors in grammar, spelling and punctuation can lead to ambiguity and confusion, or can actually give the opposite message to what you intend. Second, such errors

can give a very poor impression and can undermine professional credibility.

4 *Distinguish between fact and opinion* It is inevitable that, from time to time, we will get things wrong - we will be mistaken. It is therefore important that we do not present opinions as if they were facts. Beware of writing, for example, 'John is unlikely to cope at home' when what you really mean is 'I believe that John is unlikely to cope at home'. Presenting an opinion, even if it is a valid opinion, as if it were an undisputed fact can be very misleading and can be very problematic.

5 *Remember that clarity is more important than style* Some people try very hard to make what they write sound very impressive. For example, by using technical terms or a very formal style. Unfortunately, this is often at the expense of clarity. Some reports 'sound' impressive but, because its not very clear what the writer is trying to say, they are, in fact, far from impressive. It is wise, therefore, to concentrate on expressing yourself clearly - getting the message across plainly and without distortion.

6 *Draw conclusions where appropriate* Some reports are simply where you provide information but other reports require you to make recommendations - to draw conclusions. In preparing reports try to be clear about whether you are expected to make recommendations. If you are, make sure that you think carefully about what these should be and, if you feel at all unsure, talk these over with your line manager or a senior colleague.

7 *Check what you have written* You are responsible for what you have written and so it is vital that you check carefully what you have written. A missing word or the wrong word (for example, writing 'now' when you meant 'not') can significantly alter the meaning of what you write. Similarly, if you arrange to have written work typed, remember that it is your responsibility to proof-read it. Even the best typists make mistakes from time to time, and so you need to make sure that significant errors have not crept in.

EXERCISE 5.2

This exercise involves watching two (or more) people in conversation and noting the non-verbal dimension of their interactions. Consider the different aspects of non-verbal communications shown in figure 5.2. Watch carefully and see which of these aspects you can dentify and consider how these affect the communications taking place. Use the space below to make some notes.

Like exercise 5.1 this is an exercise that is best repeated a number of times rather than simply done once. This can help you develop your skills and sensitivity.

Non-verbal communication

Of course, communication is not just a matter of what we write or what we say - the non-verbal side of communication is also a very significant part of communication. That is, body language is important because it too conveys information - it can give very clear and powerful messages. And the very significant fact to note here is that, at times, there can be a contradiction between what is said and what is communicated non-verbally. For example, imagine that you are asked to do something that you are reluctant to do. You may respond by saying 'Yes' but, more significantly, your body language (your lack of eye-contact perhaps) may convey the opposite message. Usually, in such circumstances, it is the non-verbal communication that is likely to have the greater impact. There are two sets of implications that flow from this. First, in terms of your own communication, it is important to make sure that, as far as possible, what you say and what your body says are consistent and compatible. If not, you run the risk of confusing and

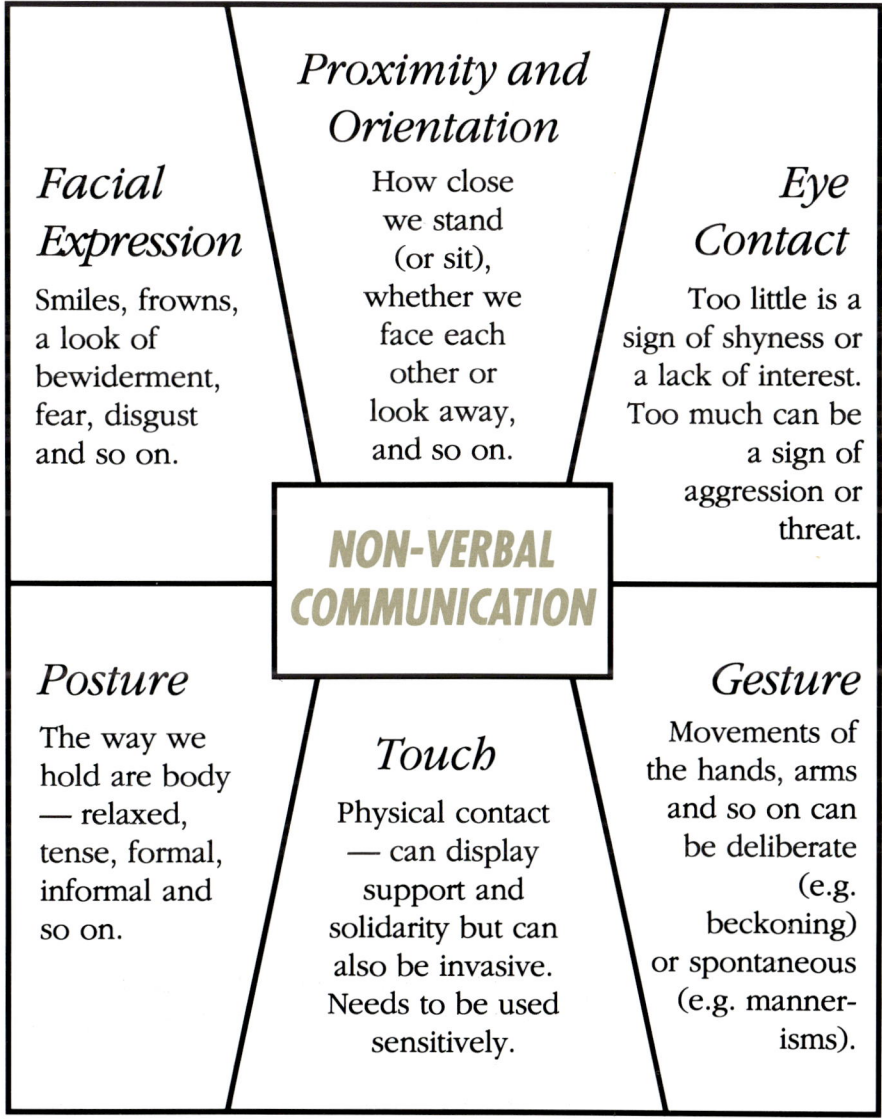

*Figure 5.2
Aspects of non-verbal
communication*

83

misleading people. Second, reading body language is an important communication skill and one well worth developing.

As Figure 5.2 shows, there are many dimensions to non-verbal communication. Understanding body language is therefore not a simple or straightforward matter. However, we do have a 'headstart' in this respect in so far as we tend to develop some degree of sensitivity to body language as a normal part of growing up. The task, therefore, is not to 'start from scratch' in learning about non-verbal behaviour but, rather, to build on the foundations we already have. This involves enhancing our sensitivity to body language by sharpening up the skills we already possess. Exercise 5.2 is designed to help with this process.

A further important point to note with regard to non-verbal communication is that it is not fixed or absolute. That is, it varies according to such factors as gender, culture and class. For example, consider such aspects as proximity and touch. How close people stand to one another and in what circumstances it is acceptable to touch - these are matters that depend very much on the people concerned in terms of what sex they are and their cultural and/or class background. For example, a handshake for people of a certain background can be a sign of friendship, whilst for others, it can be a sign of formality and distance. Sensitivity to non-verbal communication therefore needs to encompass:

- *awareness of gender issues*; for example, the danger of some aspects of body language resulting in, or being interpreted as sexual harassment;

- *ethnically-sensitive practice*; We need to be wary of offending people by disregarding cultural or religious variations in non-verbal communication;

- *respecting class differences*; A traditional criticism of social care is that it seeks to impose middle class values on working class people. We should be careful to ensure that our body language does not reinforce or exacerbate any perceived class differences.

There is no easy short-cut to achieving success in these areas. It involves getting to know the people we work with and their backgrounds. It also involves being sensitive to the way people communicate at a non-verbal level. Just as good verbal communication is premised on active listening, so too is good non-verbal communication based on 'having our eyes open' - paying attention to the significant patterns of communication arising from the non-verbal aspects of our interactions.

Conclusion

Communication skills are an important part of the value base of social care as it is through communication that people interact; it is through communication that service providers make a difference - for good or ill - to the lives and well being of service users. Good communication is an essential part of good practice and poor communication is a significant barrier to high quality social care.

As we have seen, communication is important at three levels - verbal, written and non-verbal. However, we should be wary of making the mistake of seeing these three aspects as the only ones. They provide a useful framework for understanding communication but we also need to be more flexible by looking at the specific communication needs of individuals. In short, we should be wary of losing sight of the very specific and personal nature of communication. Understanding the general patterns of communication is only the beginning and prepares the way for more advanced knowledge and skill development in terms of, for example, dealing with more complex situations where people have special communication needs or where factors such as anger or fear are to the fore. Communication is a complex and demanding subject, but it is to be hoped that this part of the pack has shown that it is also a fascinating and vitally important one.

NOTES

NOTES

NOTES

NOTES

NOTES

6

Conclusion

Conclusion

The value base of social care is an essential area of study for all staff. We cannot hope to achieve good practice in social care unless we appreciate the central role of values, particularly in terms of:

- challenging discrimination and oppression;
- maintaining confidentiality;
- promoting individuality and identity;
- ensuring effective communication.

These, then, are crucial aspects of good practice and they all reflect what is perhaps the most fundamental value of social care - that of valuing people, treating all people as important and therefore with respect and dignity. This pack can play a part in developing the skills and values we need to provide the best possible care for the people we work with. However, we should not become complacent and assume that studying this pack is all that is needed. Indeed, this pack should be seen as the beginning of the process, rather than the end of one. Promoting the value base of social care involves developing a range of skills. Skill development is a long-term process and so your studies can only help you along the way - they cannot provide you with all the answers. The task, therefore, is to carry on learning, to use the knowledge gained not as an end in itself but as steps towards future learning - part of a process of continuous professional development. So, congratulations on completing the pack. We hope you have found it useful and stimulating and well worth the hard work you have put into it. We also hope you will share our view of learning as a continuous process - one from which you will gain considerable benefit, enjoyment and pride.

7

References

References

Ahmad, B. (1990) *Black Perspectives in Social Work*, Birmingham, Venture Press.

Biestek, F. (1961) *The Casework Relationship*, London, George Allen and Unwin.
Brayne, H. and Martin, G. (1991) *Law for Social Workers*, 2nd.edn, London, Blackstone Press.
Bullock, A. and Stallybrass, O. (1977) *Dictionary of Modern Thought*, London, Fontana.

Chalton, S. and Gaskill, S. (1988) *Data Protection Law*, London, Sweet and Maxwell.
Commission for Racial Equality (CRE) (1985) *Race and Housing in Liverpool* - A Research Report, London, CRE.
Coombe, V. and Little, A. (eds) (1986) *Race and Social Work*, London, Tavistock.

Fennell, C. Phillipson, C. and Evers, H. (1988) *The Sociology of Old Age*, Milton Keynes, Open University Press.

Greater London Council (GLC) (1985) *A Charter for Lesbian and Gay Rights*, Greater London Council.

Husband, C. (1986) 'Racism, Prejudice and Social Policy', in Coombe and Little (1986).

Lorde, A. (1984) *Sister Outsider*, New York, The Crossing Press.

Oliver, M. (1983) *Social Work with Disabled People*, London, Macmillan.

Sone, K. (1991) 'Outward Bound' *Community Care, 8 August*.

Thompson, N. (1992) *Existentialism and Social Work*, Aldershot, Avebury.
Thompson, N. (1993) *Anti-Discriminatory Practice*, London, Macmillan.

Webb, R. and Tossell, D. (1991) *Social Issues for Carers*, London, Edward Arnold.

8

Guide to
Further Reading

Guide to Further Reading

Anti-Discriminatory Practice

Ahmad, B. (1990) *Black Perspectives in Social Work,* Birmingham, Venture Press.

Hanmer, J. and Statham, D. (1989) *Women and Social Work,* London, Macmillan.

Oliver, M. (1990) *The Politics of Disablement,* London, Macmillan.

Thompson, N. (1993) *Anti-Discriminatory Practice,* London, Macmillan.

Rights and Choice

Beresford, P. and Croft, S. (1993) *Citizen Involvement,* London, Macmillan.

Social Services Inspectorate (1989) *Homes are for Living In,* London, HMSO.

Social Services Inspectorate (1990) *Guidance on Standards for Residential Homes for Elderly People,* London, HMSO.

Social Services Inspectorate (1992) *Guidance on Standards for the Residential Needs of People with Learning Disabilities/Mental Handicap,* London, HMSO.

Social Services Inspectorate (1992) *Guidance on Standards for the Residential Needs of People with Specific Mental Health Needs,* London, HMSO.

Individuality and Identity

Erikson, E.H.(1977) *Childhood and Society,* London, Paladin.

Glover, J. (1988) I: *The Philosophy and Psychology of Personal Identity,* Harmondsworth, Penguin.

Gross, R.D. (1992) *Psychology,* London, Hodder and Stoughton.

Workbook 1 of Open University Course - K254 Working with Children and Young People.

Communications Skills

Crompton, M. (1990) *Attending to Children,* London, Edward Arnold.

Hargie, O. (ed.) (1986) *A Handbook of Communication Skills,* London, Routledge.

Lishman, J. (1993) *Communication,* London, Macmillan.

Petrie, P. (1989) *Communicating with Children and Adults,* London, Edward Arnold.

9

*Appendix 1
Anti-discrimination
Legislation*

Appendix 1
Anti-discrimination Legislation

The main legislation covering racial discrimination is contained within the Race Relations Acts of 1965, 1968 and 1976. Basically, the law prohibits two types of discrimination, direct and indirect:

Direct discrimination: This refers to overt and explicit discrimination on racial/ethnic grounds in terms of housing, education, employment and so on. Treating people unfairly in these areas, simply on the basis of racial or ethnic background is unlawful.

Indirect discrimination: This can be seen to apply when discrimination arises, even though this may not be direct or overt. For example, in setting particular requirements, such as a high level of fluency in the English language, employers would be excluding certain groups of people. To avoid breaking the law, any such requirements must be strictly relevant. It should also be noted that s.71 of the Race Relations Act 1976 lays a duty on local authorities to:

> *make arrangements with a view to ensuring that their various functions are carried out with due regard to the need -*
> *a. to eliminate unlawful racial discrimination; and*
> *b. to promote equality of opportunity, and good relations, between persons of different racial groups. (Brayne and Martin, 1991, p. 309).*

In addition, more recent legislation (the Children Act 1989, the NHS and Community Care Act 1990, and the Criminal Justice Act1991) emphasises the need to take account of issues of race and culture.

With regard to sex discrimination, the important statutes are the Equal Pay Act 1990, and the Sex Discrimination Act 1975. The former act makes it illegal to offer lower wages to someone on the grounds of gender. That is, the rate for the job should be the same, regardless of whether it is a man or woman in post - a measure designed to outlaw the previous practice of offering women lower rates of pay than their male counterparts. The Sex Discrimination Act 1975 makes it illegal to discriminate against someone on the grounds of their gender (or marital status). This applies to both direct and indirect discrimination as defined above.

A range of pamphlets and other materials is available from:

Commission for Racial Equality
10/12, Allington Street,
LONDON, SW1E 5EH

Equal Opportunities Commission
Overseas House,
Quay Street,
MANCHESTER, M3 3HN

*Appendix 2
The Law Relating to
Record-keeping*

Appendix 2
The Law Relating to Record-keeping

The two main pieces of legislation relating to record-keeping are; The Data Protection Act 1984 and The Access to Personal Records Act 1987.

The Data Protection Act 1984 relates to information stored on computer. It requires individuals or organisations who hold personal data to be registered with an official 'Registrar', set up specifically for this purpose. The main purpose of the legislation is to safeguard electronically stored information and to regulate access to it. The registered person is required to specify the purpose of maintaining the data (eg a company holding a list of customers), who has access to the information, the nature of the information and so on. It is an offence for an unregistered person to hold personal data and a registered person must:

> *restrict his holdings of personal data so that they conform
> with his registered particulars (Section 5(2)), and specifically
> he must not:*
> *(a) hold personal data of any description other than those
> specified in his entry on the register;*
> *(b) hold or use any personal data for any purpose other than
> a purpose described in his entry;*
> *(c) obtain any personal data, or information to be contained
> in such data, to be held by him from any source which is not
> described in his entry;*
> *(d) disclose any personal data held by him to any person
> who is not described in the entry; or*
> *(e) directly or indirectly transfer any personal data to any
> country or territory outside the United Kingdom other than
> one named or described in the entry. (Chalton and Gaskill,
> 1988, p. 1015)*

Registered persons must allow individuals to have access to the information held about them and, where this information is found to be false or inaccurate, the individual has a right to insist that it is erased or amended. For further information on this act, see Chalton and Gaskill (1988) or contact the person in your organisation who is responsible for computer records.

The Access to Personal Records Act 1987 requires Social Services Departments and other holders of personal data (other than health records) to make the information available to the individual concerned if he or she requests this. However, there are other factors which need to be taken into account:

1 'Third party' information is excluded, that is confidential information from other people such as doctors, teachers and so on.

2 Information which may be harmful to the individual or his/her family can be withheld.

3 Individuals can only see information about themselves and not about other members of their family.